How I Beat Cancer
Dr. Diana Hardy

Published by
Diana Hardy International
17503 La Cantera Parkway, Suite 104-193,
San Antonio, TX 78257
contactus@dianahardy.org

ISBN-13: 978-0794661230
ISBN-10: 0974661236

Dedication

It is with great pleasure and admiration that I dedicate this book to my Hero, the Lord Jesus Christ. He healed me! Every time I replay that day in my mind it brings tears to my eyes. I know without a doubt if He did not help me, I would not have been here to enjoy my first grandchild, Layla. All the glory and honor to Him forever.

Contents

Acknowledgment

I dedicate this offering (a piece of my heart) to my staff who are powerful vessels and wonderful human beings. Three people God gave to me so that I would see and feel His love here on earth. I called them my YES team; they were there when I needed someone to take care of both my physical and emotional needs. They are three diamonds in my crown, and even though many years have gone by, they are still here with me, doing the precious work of our Lord Jesus the Christ. They are the epitome of what it means to be a true servant of God! I will never forget their commitment and dedication to the vision that God gave me. I will love them always; they are engraved in my heart.

Preface

It's been over a decade since that day when I heard those frightful words "colon cancer" at the age of thirty-nine. Suddenly I had an epiphany that I was at a crossroad in my life. Arising out of this is a great revelation that every human being should experience, and that is to learn the importance of his/her own decisions and choices, and, more importantly, that there is someone who loves you more than you love yourself, and that is God. Yes, God made doctors and medicine, but He alone is our healer. That day God gave me the gift of life once again. While one physician diagnosed me with cancer, the other One gave me the cure.

CHAPTER 1

Only Thirty Nine Years Old

It's a shame. You're only thirty-nine years old." As I opened my eyes, these were the life-draining words I heard while coming up out of anesthesia in the recovery room. The doctor had just informed me that I had a tumor in my large intestines. And the biopsy showed that it was colon cancer. As I sit here now and think about those words that were said to me, I am so grateful that I did not own those words. I did not own that diagnosis. I am grateful I stood on the Word of God. Because when that gastroenterologist said that to me, two of my church staff members were standing with me, one on each side of the bed, and the doctor was exiting the room. Not the best bedside manner.

But when he made that comment to me, I heard God speak so strongly to me and say: "You don't have cancer."

Now I was faced with this dilemma. I instantaneously had to make a decision on whose report I was going to believe. Was I going to believe God or the doctor? I chose to immediately believe God. And because of that I am here to write this story. I told the doctor, "Doctor, I don't have cancer." After I said it the first time, he started to tell me about how he was going to refer me to an oncologist. I said to him again, "I don't have cancer."

He said, "Why do you say that? I've been a gastroenterologist for twenty years. I know that this tumor is cancerous."

And I said, "Because God just told me that I don't have cancer." And he just looked at me with this "She's in denial" look and walked out the room.

I received this diagnosis three days before Christmas 2002. I'll never forget it as long as I live. It changed my life. I got dressed and was discharged and left the hospital. On the way riding home, I guess, like any human being, I wanted to have a pity party. But when God gave me back my life after that doctor had tried to snatch it, along with His words came a sense of peace that was so powerful that every time I tried to go on a pity party (and I did try), I just could not. You want to feel sorry for yourself. After all, I had three children to think about. But I couldn't even cry. I couldn't convince myself even for a moment that I had cancer. I couldn't receive those words because I had heard God. And when I told my children about the diagnosis, they brushed it off. My oldest son said matter-of-factly, "Oh, Mom, you don't have cancer." They just wouldn't receive it; they were so sure. I was so blessed that year. That is the greatest blessing besides my salvation that God has given me.

I want to share my story of how I defeated cancer. God even proved to me in a dream that He restored my life. This dream happened shortly after my surgery. One night I dreamed that I died and as soon as my spirit left my body, God said, "Don't be afraid, I am here." Then He said, "I am sending you back." During the time He was speaking, all I could see was darkness. I saw no image, but I heard His voice; it was so reassuring and gentle—very fatherly. I am proud to say that it is now ten years later exactly. And I am healthy and full of life. I never needed chemo or radiation. And I am totally convinced that I am here because I stood on the word of God and believed what He said and refused to be moved.

Most people are not aware of the fact that God wants to have a conversation with them. I used to be one of those people who thought that He took requests and that He would never respond to us in an audible voice. But those of us who have taken the time to cultivate an honest relationship with Him are truly amazed that not only will He speak in our language to us, but His voice has a very soothing and tender nature to it. Of course, there are many ways God speaks to us; it can be by sending us strong impression, a knowing, a dream, or through somebody else. God has manifold ways of getting our attention. But one thing I want you to know is that sickness doesn't come from God. There is a scripture that says:

"Therefore, put on every piece of God's armor so you will be able to resist the enemy in the time of evil. Then, after the battle you will still be standing firm. Stand your ground, putting on the belt of truth and the body armor of

God's righteousness" (Ephesians 6:13–14, New Living Translation (NLT)).

Once I went home from the hospital. I continued to gird myself up, dressing myself with God's truth. I did have to have surgery. They removed a foot of my colon and a nasty tumor of which I had a color picture. It really did look horrible. I went home that day determined that I was going to stand and hold on to what God told me, because one thing I knew is that God is not a liar. He said it specifically in His word:

"God is not a man, so he does not lie. He is not human, so he does not change his mind. Has he ever spoken and failed to act? Has he ever promised and not carried it through?" (Numbers 23:19, NLT).

I made that my mantra. During my process I found a little book called *Healed of Cancer* by Dodie Olsteen. A very powerful little book! She used forty scriptures as her medicine every day while she was coming through metastatic liver cancer. God healed her, and it's been over twenty years. She's vibrant and she still is preaching the gospel of Jesus Christ and sharing her story all over the world.

I want to say to you that God made man and He ordained medicine, so I am not knocking cancer treatments. I do think it is a personal decision each person has to make for himself. I do know that the doctor is not a healer. He treats patients, but God is our healer. So if you want to be healed, you need to go to God. Don't leave Him out of the equation. Don't rely only on medicine, but rely on God. I can't emphasize that enough.

I did have surgery. There may be people who wouldn't have done that. After I got home and started to read that book and talk to God about what the doctor said, He reassured me, and I found every healing scripture I could in the Bible. What I did to help me go through those times when the spirit of deception would come, the enemy, and would try to suggest to my mind that I wasn't healed, I would take 8½-by-11-inch copy paper and make a sign with the scriptures on it and tape it to the walls all around me in my bedroom. One of the scriptures was from Exodus, where God says,

". . . .I am the God that healeth thee." (Exodus 15:26 King James Version (KJV))

Another scripture I had was

"He came and healed them and delivered them from their destruction" (Psalm 107:20 KJV).

I read them every day, over and over. Like Mrs. Olsteen, I took those scriptures as my daily medicine. I thanked God. I was persecuted, but I was able to stand in my healing that God had given to me. I realized this was a resurrection for me. It was three days before Christmas, and the doctor sent the biopsy to the pathologist informing me that it would take five days before I would get the results. Suffice it to say Christmas was challenging that year. After the holiday, the doctor called and told me that they could not say it was cancer; they weren't 100 percent sure. He would need me to clean out again and come back for another biopsy.

Full of dread, I conceded, knowing that I would have another five days to wait. I know some of you right now are waiting on a diagnosis, and it is excruciating. I encourage you to start talking to God right now, no matter where you are. The hospital, nursing home, in a bar, on a farm, it doesn't matter. Start talking to God about it right now. Open up and speak from your heart. And tell God about it. Give it all you've got—after all, this means your life and the quality thereof. If it's sickness in your body, whether it is life threatening or not, ask God to heal you. He said in His word,

"Yet you do not have because you do not ask (James 4:2 New King James Version (NKJV)).

And please just don't ask once. Jesus gives an illustration in Luke 11:5-13 (KJV) of how we ought to ask God for what we desire:

"Then, teaching them more about prayer, he used this story: 'Suppose you went to a friend's house at midnight, wanting to borrow three loaves of bread. You say to him, 'A friend of mine has just arrived for a visit, and I have nothing for him to eat.' And suppose he calls out from his bedroom, 'Don't bother me. The door is locked for the night, and my family and I are all in bed. I can't

help you.' But I tell you this—though he won't do it for friendship's sake, if you keep knocking long enough, he will get up and give you whatever you need because of your shameless persistence. 'And so I tell you, keep on asking, and you will receive what you ask for. Keep on seeking, and you will find. Keep on knocking, and the door will be opened to you. For everyone who asks, receives. Everyone who seeks, finds. And to everyone who knocks, the door will be opened. 'You fathers—if your children ask for a fish, do you give them a snake instead? Or if they ask for an egg, do you give them a scorpion? Of course not! So if you sinful people know how to give good gifts to your children, how much more will your heavenly Father give the Holy Spirit to those who ask him.'"

Another important decision and step that you must make is crucial to God saving your life and you regaining your health. It is to give your life to the Lord. You need to receive the gift of salvation before you can really expect God to give you the divine healing that the Bible says is the children's bread (Matthew 15:16). This promise is for God's children. Just say, "Lord, I invite You in my life, Lord Jesus. I believe You died on the cross for me. I believe You were buried and rose three days later that I might have a chance at eternal life. I invite You to be my Lord and Master." If you say those words from your heart, the Bible says that those who call on the name of the Lord shall be saved (Romans 10:13). That's just one of the benefits for those who call and invite Him into their life, their heart. Now when you say "Be my Lord and Master," you are inviting Him into every aspect of your life, making Him master of everything you own, from your body to your bank account to your children. *Everything!* You no longer have the ownership of your body or life, He does.

Cancer is a destructive disease which originates from a demonic spirit that infiltrates and attacks the lives of millions of people every day, robbing them of their hope and happiness. You are going to need someone that is more powerful than that demonic spirit. And that person is Jesus the Christ. When you have Jesus, you have the Father. The Bible says,

" . . . .no man cometh unto the Father but by me." (John 14:6KJV).

That's what Jesus said. So if you have embraced a religion of any kind other than the Gospel of Jesus Christ, I want you to know you will not be saved by it. There is only one true God, so you need to renounce any religion you are currently embracing to embrace Jesus Christ as your Lord and you will have a miraculous change in your life. That's the beginning. That's what you need to do to start your divine healing.

You are now a new creature in Christ (2Corinthians 5:17), part of the Kingdom of God, joint heirs with Christ Jesus (Romans 8:17). You have just been adopted into the family of God. Now God will come into that situation you are being confronted with.

Another thing you need to do is decide to trust God. Either you are going to trust the doctor or trust God. That doesn't mean you don't use modern medicine if that's what you desire to do. But you must ultimately believe God's Word and take His direction. Confess to yourself and other people. Once you have prayed about it and are convinced that God has heard you, you have to receive healing by faith. The difficult part comes in trusting that *you are healed*, especially when you body is displaying symptoms of a sickness. Tell people *you are healed* even if your body is currently in pain or the tumor is still there. As you confess it and believe in your heart that you are healed, that tumor will disintegrate. The Bible says,

"For as he thinks within himself, so he is" (Proverbs 23:7, New American Standard Bible (NASB)).

As you trust God that you are healed, divine healing will be released to your body and your body will come into agreement with the Word and with what you believe. Now I am not saying it will be easy to stand and not waiver. That's why I am going to give you some suggestions and tell you how I kept myself immersed in that. I took those scriptures I told you about earlier and put them all around my room. Whatever room you spend the most time in is where you need to have them.

I want you to know God is a savior. He will save you day after day after day. As I lay in that bed, I was still in pain. So I opted for the surgery and spent eight days in the hospital. It was horrible. When they remove a tumor from your colon, they split you from the top of your

19

stomach to the bottom. And then they cut out a foot of my colon. No one told me I would wake up with a tube down my throat. I wasn't prepared for that mentally, and that really messed with me to the extent that I didn't even want anyone to visit me. One of my staff members had to be there with me the whole time while I was on morphine, which was approximately four or five days.

The doctor explained to me what happens when a surgeon operates on the colon. He stated that because the colon is a muscle, when you cut it, it stops working. So they had to insert a tube that would remove the fluids that my stomach was making. So I had to endure that. I did not really feel up to talking to my kids or any of my family members. I became depressed.

The doctor said they couldn't remove the tube until I passed gas. The passing of gas would tell the doctor that my colon (a muscle) was working again. He encouraged me by telling me that usually it takes three days for it to resume its activity, but by the third day there was still no sign of activity, so we waited another two days. By then he was perplexed, so he threw his hands up and decided to remove the tube. Thank God the muscle was working. While I was on the morphine, I had a little hallucination. But I stood on God's Word that I was healed. I went home to recover.

The year before my surgery, God had instructed me in prayer to stop eating meat. Because I love God so much, He didn't have to explain to me why I needed to do what He said. I fully understood that I was made for His good pleasure (Revelation 4:11). Because He is my Creator, He can do with me what He pleases. He has the right to tell me how to live, what to do, and when. Obeying God is how you show you love and trust Him. And you can't know what to do or even what is required of you if you don't first establish a relationship with Him.

I stopped eating meat, although it was a struggle at first. I would stop, but then I would go eat a hamburger or some chicken. But I'd always talk to God and tell Him how much I was struggling to do what He said. He gave me the strength and I stopped. So it had been about a good year that I had stopped eating meat before I got my diagnosis.

I thank God. We often take for granted how much God takes care of us. Every day we wake up because God calls our name. If He doesn't call your name, you don't wake up. That's a special kind of care that no one else can provide. This is the epitome of love to me, that God is so careful over us that He wakes us up every day and gives us His strength so that we are able to get out of bed and carry on what we are supposed to do every day.

I read God's Word over and over concerning healing, as well as all of the supporting scriptures in His word. I have taken the liberty to list forty scriptures in the back of this book to help facilitate the healing that you need.

Post-surgery, I spent thirty days in bed, still in pain. I was a little, to say the least, distraught. I thought once I had the surgery that I would be good as new in a week and be able to start to resume some of my activities. It was January 2003—what a way to start the new year off.

Per doctors' orders, I couldn't lift anything, which didn't matter so much because I could only walk from the bed to the bathroom anyway. I was so weak. My staff brought my food and stayed with me at my home, taking care of me the whole time. Isn't it wonderful how God will put people in your life to help you through the tough times? I became disillusioned because I was still in pain after being in bed for three weeks. I thought that I would be able to go downstairs and do some of the things I did before. But because I was still in pain in my colon, all I could do was talk to God. I told God how much I wanted to serve Him and reminded him of the promises He made to me. And I told Him how I wanted to help people and to know my assignment, what He wanted me to do. I kept reading God's word. I was the senior pastor of a church and I was anxious to resume my activities.

In my distress, I regressed and started to eat a little chicken with my lunch and dinner. I ate that for a week or two. And then I started to feel this constant pressure to urinate often. Something started pressing on my bladder. I thought, what is going on? I just had surgery two weeks ago. They had opened me up and taken out the tumor. Why did I feel this pressure? I called the doctor, who told me to go to the gynecologist.

I made an appointment to see the doctor. When I got there I had to get a vaginal ultrasound. The technician immediately noticed a large, thirteen-centimeter mass— that is the size of a newborn baby's head—in my stomach. They diagnosed it as a chocolate cyst; it was called that because it had old blood in it. Finally, when I saw that doctor, she said, "You are going to have surgery again to cut this large cyst out."

I sighed and said, "Wait a minute! I just had surgery last month. I cannot take another surgery."

She said, "Well, this is going to stay here and continue to make you uncomfortable." She asked me what I did for this to happen. I explained about being in bed for the last four weeks, and she reiterated, "You did something." She went on to say, "When they opened you up, you didn't have this. I saw the x-rays. Did you lift something?"

I emphatically said, "No. I only went to the bathroom."

Then I remembered. I did do something different. I ate a little chicken for lunch and dinner. She told me that's what did it. I was astonished by what she said. She said: "It's the kind of protein the meat is that caused the cyst to grow." That protein caused it to grow that big in only two weeks. I said, "I am really a vegetarian. I just started eating that meat because I was depressed about being in the bed so long. So if I stop eating the meat, it will go away?"

The doctor said, "It will go down some, but it's gotten too big. You need surgery right away."

I said, "Ma'am, I am a praying and God-fearing Christian woman. I need to talk to God about this." She respected my position and said she would give me a call in a couple of days. So I went home and talked to God. After talking it over with the Lord, He told me I didn't have to have the surgery. He said, "I'll take care of it."

CHAPTER 2

Faith-Real Medicine

L et me say that to this day, I regret I didn't ask God about the first surgery to remove the tumor. I didn't ask God. I don't know whether I was so traumatized that I just didn't ask Him but just went ahead and did it. I cannot give you a real reason why I chose to leave Him out of my decision.

But I can tell you this: it was the biggest mistake I have ever made. And now, after all I had been through, this time I asked God. When you know better, you do better, right? So when the doctor called two days later, I told her God said I didn't need the surgery and that He would take care of it. She chuckled a little and said, "I respect your religion, but this large mass is not going to go anywhere. You really need to reconsider." I told her, "No, I have made my decision."

So I stayed in bed. I did make the decision to stop eating chicken that day. No more flesh for me. Two years later, I went back to the same gynecologist and, as you might have guessed, the cyst was completely gone. I can't tell you when, but the pressure to urinate stopped. It just disappeared! This is another example of divinity touching humanity, a miraculous healing. The doctor said it wouldn't go completely away. But God said it would, and it did. A second time God stepped in.

Today (2012)

At forty-nine, I am alive to enjoy my granddaughter. Had I believed the doctor, I probably would not be alive. Today, I want you to grab hold of God, and don't let go! Talk to Him throughout the day. Talk yourself clear. After all, He said in his word,

"Give all your worries and cares to God, for he cares about you. (1 Peter 5:7 NLT).

Every time you start to feel fear or grief, talk to God. If you feel like you want to give up, get His Word, the

Bible, and find the promises that He made to those who love Him. Don't let those feelings of despair creep into your mind. Go to *Bible Gateway*, plug in the word "healing," and pray and mediate on those healing scriptures. Get a Bible and start to read how God healed others and how they used their faith to overcome their obstacles. Just start reading the synoptic Gospels, Matthew, Mark, and Luke. Read how he healed blind Bartemaeus (John 9:1-15) and the child with epilepsy (Mark 9:14-29); the man that was lame who was over forty years old (Acts 4); how He healed the woman with the issue of blood (Matthew 9:20) and the woman who was bent over for eighteen years, and she stood up (Luke 13:10-17). The Apostle Paul was blind for three days and God healed him (Acts 9).

God said that He does not change (Hebrews 13:8). It doesn't matter what anyone else says. If you want to live, Jesus was talking about you when He said:

"The thief does not come except to steal, and to kill, and to destroy. I have come that you may have life and that you may have it more abundantly." (John 10:10 NKJV).

God is not finished with you. He's deeply and passionately in love with you.

That's why this booklet has come into your hands. Don't you dare give up! Take these prescriptions. I am just telling you the meat of my story—something you can grab hold of to save your life right now. I want to make myself available to you. You can e-mail me if you have any questions. If I can help you on your road to recovery, please feel free to write to me. This is the reason why I am living, to help others who are going through a battle. He saved me, so that He can save you. Isn't that precious? Imagine how much He loves you.

We don't know each other, but I know you are out there, millions of you. We have an enemy of our souls who came to steal, kill, and destroy (John 10:10). He is trying to steal your time, your love, and most of all your joy; time to love and be with your family and live. If you feel you are by yourself, you are not. I am with you. My heart is with you. It is my heartfelt desire that you live and love again. Start by letting the Lord Jesus Christ love on you day by day. He will do that.

*"When your mother and father have forsaken you, then
God will lift you up." (Psalm 27:10 KJV).*

God is going to teach you how to walk and talk with
Him. Talk to God daily from your heart. You may have
decided to take chemo and you don't have insurance. This
is your prescription. Start talking to God; ask Him to heal
you, which will be for His glory but your story. Don't give
up after you've prayed; just believe that you have received
your healing and it will manifest. Healing occurs the
moment you ask God for it and believe. So, in other words,
it is already done in the spirit. Sometimes people will pray
and the healing manifests immediately; other times it is
progressive.

A few years ago, I got sick and the doctor could not
figure out what was wrong with me. I told him my
symptoms. He thought it was a sinus infection, as that was
where much of the problem was. When I would get up, I
would get dizzy after a few minutes. So the doctor began
to treat me with antibiotics, nasal sprays, and liquid syrups.
But I continued to get sicker. He was making house visits
and thought that I would probably be sick a few days.

I ended up being confined to bed for ten weeks, and no matter what he gave me, it would not get better. He had already put me on prednisone, which wasn't working. The doctor scratched his head and said, "I don't know what to do!" after a while. Thank God I was praying the whole time and talking to the Lord, asking Him to heal me. Because I was confined to the bed, I had nothing but time to pray, and I did, for everybody and everything.

One day when I was in that bed, I felt a presence come and hover over the end of my bed. At first I thought it was an angel that God had sent with healing mercies for me, but after a while I knew it was not an angel, but the Holy Spirit Himself. It felt dark and foreboding, serious yet loving at first, but as I started to recognize and speak to Him, I felt assured but cautious. He came to me and listened and talked. I asked questions and He answered.

My walk with God changed as a result of that holy visitation. The Holy Spirit said that He would heal me, and He did very shortly thereafter. My friends had grown very concerned that my restoration was taking so long. But I was hopeful; I believed God, and if you want to be well again, you must, too.

Emphatically believe God. Don't just let others pray for you; pray continually for yourself as well. You are going to have to stand on your healing, believe it, and tell others what God has done for you even before it manifests in your physical body. In other words, you will have already received it in spirit, and once you believe, it is already done. You already have it. Just hold on to it. Tell people even though it may make you look crazy. This is how you are going to get your healing. Make sure you surround yourself with those who can believe with you and not confess anything other than your healing. The Bible says that

"without faith it is impossible to please God" (Hebrews 11:6 KJV).

You have to have faith in what He tells you, and do it and continue to do it until it manifests in your physical body. Do not allow anyone to talk you out of it. Get all negative people out of your space. It worked for me, and this same formula will work no matter what your situation is. It doesn't matter what the diagnosis is or what state you are in or where you came from. This will work for anybody, as long as he or she follows the steps outlined in this book.

Andrew Murray, one of the great generals of God, said: "Healing by means of remedies shows us the power of God in nature, but it does not bring us into living and direct contact with Him." (from *Divine Healing* by Andrew Murray).

The idea to write to you was given to me by God; I can't take credit for it. Let's give credit where it is due. So if God heals you, tell everyone what He has done for you.

He deserves all the honor and glory this brings. It speaks to His credibility as a Healer and a Savior! I fully expect to hear the success stories that will come from this. I am believing in God with you for your healing. Shoot me an e-mail and I will stand in faith with you. The Bible says when two touch and agree on anything, it will be done by the Father (Matthew 18:19). I touch and agree with you right now if you need healing in your body. I love you.

You are probably thinking, "How could you love me, Diana? You don't even know me." Throughout my twenty-plus years with God, I have asked Him for love to love His people with. All God cares about are His people. I was on the Number 1 train in New York City on my way home, and I was talking to God in my head.

And all of a sudden, He said: "I am in love with my people."

I knew I heard him, but I said, "You mean you love them."

He said: "No, I am in love with them."

God wants intimacy. And the person He wants to reveal Himself to is you. He is offering you a chance to see into Him, to be transparent (into-me-see…intimacy). Unlike so many of us who are afraid to open up and let people see who we really are, God doesn't have any fear. In fact, the Bible states,

"Perfect love casts out all fear" (1 John 4:18 KJV).

Meditate on this scripture and ask God for His perfect love. It will protect you every day.

He Sent You a Love Letter!

He started His pursuit of you by offering you a sixty-six book love letter (The Bible) to reveal His personality and how He thinks and feels about you.

There's a story in the book of Samuel where Israel was asking for a king because they wanted to be like the surrounding countries. Up until that time, God had been their king. So the people told the prophet Samuel to give them a king. Samuel was grieved, but he went to God and told Him what their request was. God told Samuel they are not rejecting you, they are rejecting Me! (1 Kings 8). So God has feelings!

Always remember God has feelings. He loves and cares, laughs, and is very concerned about the things that go on with you. That's why we have all those same components in us—because God made us in His image.

Remember the second biopsy I got? Well, when it came back, there was no cancer. I told the doctor with all the love I could muster, "Do you remember I told you I didn't have cancer?"

He smiled and said, "Have a good weekend, Ms. Hardy."

But this had to happen so I could tell my story. And this doctor now knows there is a God that sits high but looks low (Psalm 138:6). Whatever God says, He has the power to make it come to pass. And He will perform.

Spiritual Espionage

At the time that I was writing this, I had a considerable amount of weight to lose. I have lost a substantial amount of weight, and all because of God. For most of my life, I have been overweight. You wouldn't have known it growing up because I was a skinny kid. Then somewhere after puberty, I started to slowly gain weight. My mother was a full-figured woman, so obesity ran in my family.

One evening, I was talking to God while getting ready to go to bed about the promise and commitment He had made to me. I asked Him to help me lose the weight. I quoted a size to Him, to which He offered me a solution. He told me to *walk*, as simple as that. And I am happy to report that

He's keeping His promise as we speak. He told me to let go of that sorcery.

And I said, with shock on my face, "God, what sorcery?"

Very clearly He said: *"Fear."*

Well, that was an eye opener for me. I know what fear is, or should I say that I defined fear as the thing which makes us afraid to go after what we want to do or accomplish. What I didn't realize is that fear is a very diabolical strategy. There are not many people in this entire world that don't have some kind of fear in their life.

Imagine you live across the street from a neighbor and that person has been living there for years now. Every morning your neighbor has been waving and smiling at you. But you've really never had the opportunity to have a conversation with each other. Yet, he/she is always smiling and from all outward appearances is very friendly.

Imagine if you found out that all that time, the neighbor who lived across from you really didn't like you. Or, even more so, that he/she was very jealous of you.

Never would you have guessed that he/she felt that way about you. After all, he/she was never once cold or unfriendly. But you discovered that his/her disdain and jealousy for you had grown over the years and your neighbor had come to dislike you to the point of hatred.

I know that seems like something you don't understand. Why would your neighbor hate you? Perhaps you live in a nicer house or you drive an expensive car. From all outward appearances, you look like you have a better life. Maybe you have a spouse and that person doesn't. Maybe you have children and that person's children have left. There can be so many reasons people become jealous. But just as your neighbor didn't like you all these years and was jealous, Satan is jealous, and he hates you with a passion.

He is the enemy of your life. He wants your very existence to be destroyed, and the only thing stopping him is God, the One who created you and is in love with you. The reason He is stopping your enemy is because you are His prize possession and He has a purpose and an exciting plan for your life. He is excited about helping you to become all that He made you to be. Or you're the prodigal son or daughter (Luke 15) that needs to come back to God so He can love you and make you whole and happy until you are blessed, and so He can show His great power and admiration through how He treats you, getting involved in everything you invite Him into.

I gave you this analogy so that you can begin to understand how your enemy operates. He too is invisible!

Satan is furious at God's determination to love you. He has already been condemned. His judgment has taken place; God said he's going to hell, a lake of fire, with all the other demons and angels that followed him when he decided to lead a rebellion against God (Revelation 19:20).

God does not look kindly on rebellion, just as any other good parent wouldn't. It creates a ripple effect in the lives of those who participate in it, and eventually there will be repercussions. Any good parent would shell out some discipline on a child that continues to be rebellious. If your child is putting himself/herself in harm's way, you have to do whatever you can to get that child out of harm's way. Sometimes you have to intervene. That's what God does. He is the perfect example of a good parent. One of the reasons why God gave us parents is to reveal to us in the natural world what He is to us spiritually.

Scripture says,

"For God did not give us a spirit of fear, but of power, and of love, and of a sound mind" (2 Timothy 1:7KJV).

In other words, He gave us three things that will offset anything that comes against us. If we allow those things to permeate our mind and our being, they will offset what is going to come against us. He didn't give us fear, He gave us love. Perfect love casts out fear. He gave us power and a sound mind. A sound mind is self-discipline. That's what that means.

So if you have these three, you will have the core strength you need in order to live a successful and satisfying life. Your desire will be to extol God while building a relationship with Him that needs continued growth so that you can get the wisdom and direction you need. That's food for thought.

If you are battling with fear, taking the necessary steps to help free yourself is vital to your restoration. You will need guidance from someone who has already accomplished what you are trying to attain. A mentor that can help you would be appropriate.

CHAPTER 3

The Salt- Forgiveness

I would be remiss if I didn't discuss with you a very important, pertinent topic that has been instrumental in much of the degradation of mankind, and that is unforgiveness. People don't think it's necessary to discuss this topic. Quite the contrary, unforgiveness should be a hot topic in every household. People don't put a high value on talking about unforgiveness and perpetuating the truth about it.

There are so many people today who claim kingdom citizenship and read the Word of God but do not value or exercise the commandment of God to forgive each other in their lives. God made it crystal clear in His Word, no matter what translation you get, that if you don't forgive your brother, God will not forgive you (Matthew 18:21-35).

Let me repeat that again. If you don't forgive others of their sins and trespasses, then God is not going to forgive you. That's plain and clear. So those are God's thoughts and feelings about that, which means that when you do something, knowingly or unknowingly, or when you make a mistake that causes a problem for someone else and you want to be forgiven by God, He is going to look and see if there is any unforgiveness in your life for anybody, no matter what that person did. If it is there, that unforgiveness will become a barrier between you and the forgiveness *you need* for mistakes and sins. I hope that is painfully clear.

Another problem that unforgiveness presents is that it opens the door for satanically induced problems like fear and sickness to apprehend you. Consider this from a natural perspective. When you won't forgive somebody, it's like building an iron wall. On one side of the wall lives your hurt, and on the other is the person who created it.

The thing about a wall is, nothing gets in, but nothing gets out either. That same wall will keep you from sharing the better parts of you, which are what's in your heart. And unforgiveness, if allowed to stay in your heart, will slowly yet subtly start to control your actions and reactions to others. It will steal areas of your life. Steal your time. And the hope that you do have will begin draining and fear will replace it. Fear of letting someone else into your heart will attack your mind. You may worry that if you let that person in, they might just hurt you, too. Unforgiveness is dangerous to your well-being and should not be embraced or allowed to live inside of you.

You were made to be nurtured and then endeavor to nurture others. Start by forgiving everyone who hurt you. It doesn't matter what these others did. Don't let the spirit of unforgiveness take authority and have power over you. Ideally, because we are imperfect humans, we ought to forgive. If you are struggling to let go of someone else's trespass, ask God to help you forgive. Your heart is too delicate; it was made for love and passion and other good things. Wisdom, knowledge, and power want to occupy your heart. Let them have their way. Invite them into every area of your life. Remember, if you don't forgive the person, God won't forgive you.

If you have been asking God in prayer for healing and deliverance from whatever is ailing you, if you are sick in your body, or if it is mental health issues, whatever it is for you, your family, or a friend, it will not happen until you forgive. Unforgiveness blocks your blessings. So it is somewhat fruitless to ask God to heal this cancer, leukemia, or whatever the condition is if you will not forgive those who hurt you, no matter what they did. On the other hand, forgiveness is like salt. It will preserve your life and free you up for the blessings God wants to pour into life.

I want to share with you something that I was teaching on recently to the members of my congregation.

My intention was to help them to see the monuments that they have built in their lives over the years. In fact, almost all of us can identify with this. If you can remember something that someone said or did to you and you are still holding against them, you haven't forgiven them.

Instead, you left a monument behind, a marker that you put in place and every time you think of what that person said or did, the pain returns and you revisit all the ugly feelings you experienced just like when it first happened.

Some of us have so many monuments that we obtained over the years, it is no wonder that we feel burdened down most of the time. Maybe you are one of those people who will not allow yourself to experience joy or happiness for fear of being hurt again. The final result is bitterness, which is fertile soil for sickness of the heart, mind and body.

As painful as it may be, please take the necessary steps to alleviate yourself of the monuments in your life that lead to unforgiveness.

Don't focus on the bad experiences; tear down the emotional monuments that you erected to remind yourself of what happen to you. Have a heartfelt conversation with God about those areas. Ask Him to heal the hurt involved. Remember God is in your corner, He is for you.

Also, if you have someone that you can trust to talk about it to, do it. Getting it out of you will open you up to the process of healing.

PS: On a more positive note, once the process begins and you start to see the power of God operating in your life (ex. Healing, restoration, freedom, etc) make sure you set markers/monuments in those places to remind you what God did for you. Tell everyone who will listen how God visited your life. These are monuments that will reveal to you the unshakeable, unchangeable love has in His Heart toward you.

First you ask yourself, are you willing to forgive? Then, when you go to God, say: "I am willing; help me to forgive that person for what he/she did to me." I grew up in a household where my mother was the dominant parent.

My father was very easygoing. They were married for forty-six years until the day he died of prostate cancer at sixty-nine years old. My mother did so many things to me that were really somewhat unforgivable. I was verbally and physically abused, so I held that against her. I was so hurt by some of the things she did, and I felt justified in holding it against her for so many years, to the point where I was so angry with her, so disappointed with her as a mother, that I told people in school my mother was dead. I made up a mother from another country. A whole different nationality.

I carried that on for some years because I was angry and hurt and I held unforgiveness for her. And, as a result, sickness, anger, and low self-esteem ravished me. When I came to God I was twenty-nine years old. I was serious about God. I needed Him. So I ran to the church to find Him. I was captivated by what the preacher said. That's how God reached out to me. And I emphatically fell in love with God, and my love has grown deeper as the years go by.

As time went on, I went to the Bible Church of Christ, a deliverance ministry. I made the decision that whatever was in me or my life that wasn't the will God, I wanted it out! I was desperate to know what His plan for my life was. I had wandered in the wilderness long enough, and I had enough pain in me to destroy the lives of a few people. I went up for prayer and I told them I wanted to be delivered from anything that was not pleasing to God.

And as I was standing there, the Lord said to me, "When are you going to forgive your mother?" At that time, I didn't know what one thing had to do with the other. But it had everything to do with it, because that was the thing that was blocking me.

When God pulls on your heart, listen to Him. Don't ignore those feelings or His voice. Whether you hear Him audibly or you have a strong feeling, it doesn't matter. He has so many ways of talking to you. Be careful how you respond to Him. Tell Him the truth; don't tell Him a lie. If you tell Him a lie you made up for people, it won't work. He knows everything. He's omniscient. He knows all!

What I said to Him was, "God, I will forgive her if you help me." From that moment, it meant that the help was present right then. It meant I was able to do it right then. And from that moment, I forgave her. I made the choice in my heart.

What am I saying to you? It's a choice; that's where you start. I chose to let go of the trespass I had against her. When God spoke to me, I realized what He said was necessary for me to continue in my relationship with Him.

And from that moment I forgave her. And doors opened up. The weight that I had carried for twenty years just dropped off. Words cannot describe how I felt.

Imagine how one choice, one decision, will either keep you in sickness, bondage, and fear or set you free from all of those. These steps I have given you are very important for your emotional and physical healing for you to live the kind of life you deserve: a happy, fear-free, productive life, a prosperous life. The Apostle John said,

"Above all, beloved, I wish that you may prosper and be in good health. And that's my prayer for you."(3 John 1:2 KJV).

Father, in the Name of Jesus, I thank You for the opportunity to write this manual, to share with Your children, my sisters and brothers, wisdom You have given me that has helped me to live an abundant life and has set me free from fear and sickness and has blessed me tremendously.

I pray for every soul, every heart, every person who reads this book and shares it with someone else, be it a friend, family, or someone else. I pray that You would save this person if they are not saved. I claim this person for the kingdom of God and for Your righteousness. And I ask that You would visit them today. I thank You for loving them. And whatever they are asking You for, if it be Your will and in Your word, I stand in agreement with this person, God. I touch and agree with them on their request before you.

I love You and I thank You.

In Jesus' Name, amen.

CHAPTER 4

Forty Healing Scriptures

He said, "If you will listen carefully to the voice of the LORD your God and do what is right in his sight, obeying his commands and keeping all his decrees, then I will not make you suffer any of the diseases I sent on the Egyptians; for I am the LORD who heals you."

Exodus 15:26 (NLT)

"You must serve only the LORD your God. If you do, I will bless you with food and water, and I will protect you from illness."

Exodus 23:25

And the LORD will protect you from all sickness. He will not let you suffer from the terrible diseases you knew in Egypt, but he will inflict them on all your enemies!

Deuteronomy 7:15

"Today I have given you the choice between life and death, between blessings and curses. Now I call on heaven and earth to witness the choice you make. Oh, that you would choose life, so that you and your descendants might live!"

Deuteronomy 30:19

Do not dread the disease that stalks in darkness, nor the disaster that strikes at midday.

Psalm 91:6

Let all that I am praise the LORD; with my whole heart, I will praise His holy name. Let all that I am praise the LORD; may I never forget the good things He does for me. He forgives all my sins and heals all my diseases. He redeems me from death and crowns me with love and tender mercies. He fills my life with good things. My youth is renewed like the eagle's!

Psalm 103:1–5

He sent out His word and healed them, snatching them from the door of death.

Psalm 107:20

I will not die; instead, I will live to tell what the LORD has done.

Psalm 118:17

My child, pay attention to what I say. Listen carefully to my words. Don't lose sight of them. Let them penetrate deep into your heart, for they bring life to those who find them, and healing to their whole body.

Proverbs 4:20–22

But he was pierced for our rebellion, crushed for our sins. He was beaten so we could be whole. He was whipped so we could be healed.

Isaiah 53:5

I will give you back your health and heal your wounds,"" says the LORD. "For you are called an outcast— 'Jerusalem for whom no one cares.' "

Jeremiah 30:17

Why are you scheming against the LORD? He will destroy you with one blow; he won't need to strike twice!

Nahum 1:9

Suddenly, a man with leprosy approached Him and knelt before Him. "Lord," the man said, "if You are willing, You can heal me and make me clean." Jesus reached out and touched him. "I am willing," he said. "Be healed!" And instantly the leprosy disappeared.

Matthew 8:2–3

"I tell you the truth, whatever you forbid on earth will be forbidden in heaven, and whatever you permit on earth will be permitted in heaven."

Matthew 18:18

"I also tell you this: If two of you agree here on earth concerning anything you ask, my Father in heaven will do it for you."

Matthew 18:19

Then Jesus said to the disciples, "Have faith in God. I tell you the truth, you can say to this mountain, 'May you be lifted up and thrown into the sea,' and it will happen. But you must really believe it will happen and have no doubt in your heart."

Mark 11:22–23

These miraculous signs will accompany those who believe: They will cast out demons in my name, and they will speak in new languages. They will be able to handle snakes with safety, and if they drink anything poisonous, it won't hurt them. They will be able to place their hands on the sick, and they will be healed."

Mark 16:17–18

The thief's purpose is to steal and kill and destroy. My purpose is to give you a rich and satisfying life.

John 10:10

The Spirit of God, who raised Jesus from the dead, lives in you. And just as God raised Christ Jesus from the dead, he will give life to your mortal bodies by this same Spirit living within you.

Romans 8:11

For all of God's promises have been fulfilled in Christ with a resounding "Yes!" And through Christ, our "Amen" (which means "Yes") ascends to God for His glory.

2 Corinthians 1:20

We use God's mighty weapons, not worldly weapons, to knock down the strongholds of human reasoning and to destroy false arguments. We destroy every proud obstacle that keeps people from knowing God. We capture their rebellious thoughts and teach them to obey Christ.

2 Corinthians 10:4-5

But Christ has rescued us from the curse pronounced by the law. When He was hung on the cross, He took upon Himself the curse for our wrongdoing. For it is written in the Scriptures, "Cursed is everyone who is hung on a tree." Through Christ Jesus, God has blessed the Gentiles with the same blessing He promised to Abraham, so that we who are believers might receive the promised Holy Spirit through faith.

Galatians 3:13–14

A final word: Be strong in the Lord and in His mighty power. Put on all of God's armor so that you will be able to stand firm against all strategies of the devil. For we are not fighting against flesh-and-blood enemies, but against evil rulers and authorities of the unseen world, against mighty powers in this dark world, and against evil spirits in the heavenly places. Therefore, put on every piece of God's armor so you will be able to resist the enemy in the time of evil. Then after the battle you will still be standing firm.

Ephesians 6:10–13

For God is working in you, giving you the desire and the power to do what pleases Him.

Philippians 2:13

For God has not given us a spirit of fear and timidity, but of power, love, and self-discipline.

2 Timothy 1:7

Let us hold tightly without wavering to the hope we affirm, for God can be trusted to keep His promise.

Hebrews 10:23

So do not throw away this confident trust in the Lord. Remember the great reward it brings you!

Hebrews 10:35

Jesus Christ is the same yesterday, today, and forever.

Hebrews 13:8

Are any of you sick? You should call for the elders of the church to come and pray over you, anointing you with oil in the name of the Lord. Such a prayer offered in faith will heal the sick, and the Lord will make you well. And if you have committed any sins, you will be forgiven.

James 5:14–15

He personally carried our sins in His body on the cross so that we can be dead to sin and live for what is right. By His wounds you are healed.

1 Peter 2:24

And we are confident that He hears us whenever we ask for anything that pleases Him. And since we know He hears us when we make our requests, we also know that He will give us what we ask for.

1 John 5:14–15

Dear friends, if we don't feel guilty, we can come to God with bold confidence. And we will receive from Him whatever we ask because we obey Him and do the things that please Him.

1 John 3:21–22

Dear friend, I hope all is well with you and that you are as healthy in body as you are strong in spirit.

3 John 1:2

And they have defeated him by the blood of the Lamb and by their testimony. And they did not love their lives so much that they were afraid to die.

Revelation 12:11

Not a single one of all the good promises the LORD had given to the family of Israel was left unfulfilled; everything He had spoken came true.

Joshua 21:45

"Bring all the tithes into the storehouse so there will be enough food in my temple. If you do," says the LORD of Heaven's Armies, "I will open the windows of heaven for you. I will pour out a blessing so great you won't have enough room to take it in! Try it! Put me to the test!"

Malachi 3:10

"I—yes, I alone—will blot out your sins for My own sake and will never think of them again. Let us review the situation together, and you can present your case to prove your innocence."

Isaiah 43:25-26

We know that God doesn't listen to sinners, but He is ready to hear those who worship Him and do His will.

John 9:31

These are the forty healing scriptures, in the New Living Translation, used by Dodie Olsteen from her book, *Healed of Cancer*.

God bless you. I am going to be praying for you as these books go out. I am going to pray that God both heals and restores you and that you'll be better than you were. I love you. Have an awesome life.

About the Author

Dr. Diana Hardy is founder and senior pastor of the Victory Lamp in San Antonio, Texas and CEO of Diana Hardy International. A leader and visionary, Dr. Hardy helms a multifaceted ministry that reaches beyond the walls of the church to touch the very heart of a God generation. She has accepted the divine assignment to sound the horn and call forth the God generation right now—a generation that lives in divine healing, prosperity, and irrefutable power.

Dr. Hardy holds a bachelor's in theology, a master's in business administration, and is currently working on her second doctorate in psychology. She has three loving children and a dedicated congregation. It is through the power of God and faith in His word that Dr. Hardy is alive today to see her beautiful granddaughter growing up. She now takes every opportunity to share the miracle of healing and transformation that is her life to encourage her fellow human beings.

www.ingramcontent.com/pod-product-compliance
Lightning Source LLC
Chambersburg PA
CBHW031613040426
42452CB00006B/497